MAY 29 19[illegible]

UNIV. OF MICH.
LIBRARY

616.9955
N533T

DEPARTMENT OF HEALTH

OF THE

CITY OF NEW YORK

NO. 3 TUBERCULOSIS MONOGRAPH APRIL, 1917

TUBERCULOSIS IN RELATION TO FEEBLEMINDEDNESS

BY

PETER BRYCE, M.A., M.D.

CHIEF MEDICAL OFFICER OF THE INTERIOR, AND CHIEF MEDICAL INSPECTOR OF IMMIGRATION FOR CANADA

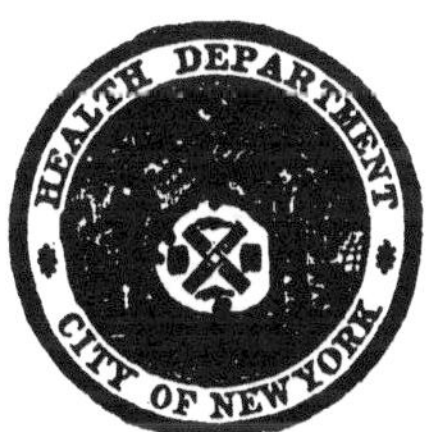

Public health is purchasable. Within natural limitations a community can determine its own death rate.

DEPARTMENT OF HEALTH

OF THE

CITY OF NEW YORK

DEPARTMENT OF HEALTH

OF THE

CITY OF NEW YORK

No. 3 TUBERCULOSIS MONOGRAPH APRIL, 1917

TUBERCULOSIS IN RELATION TO FEEBLEMINDEDNESS

BY

PETER BRYCE, M.A., M.D.

CHIEF MEDICAL OFFICER OF THE INTERIOR, AND CHIEF MEDICAL INSPECTOR OF IMMIGRATION FOR CANADA

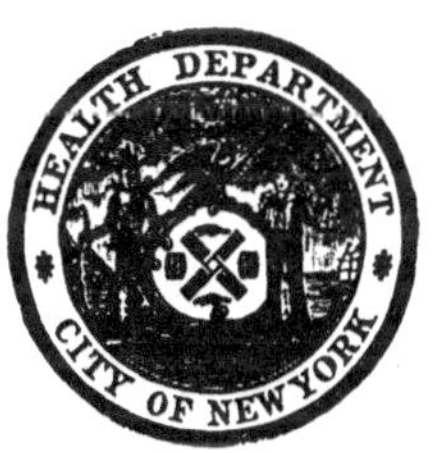

Public health is purchasable. Within natural limitations a community can determine its own death rate.

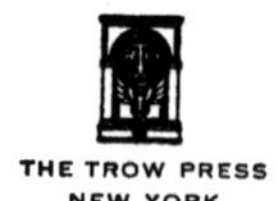

THE TROW PRESS
NEW YORK

TUBERCULOSIS IN RELATION TO FEEBLEMINDEDNESS*

By PETER BRYCE, M. A., M. D.,

Chief Medical Officer of the Interior, and Chief Medical Inspector of Immigration for Canada

I am quite aware that my personal opportunities for collecting information are not such as to entitle me to express any dogmatic conclusions on the subject I have chosen to talk about for a few moments, and yet it is perhaps true that owing to my position as Chief Medical Inspector of Immigration for Canada, I have had some phases of so many mental and physical conditions brought to my attention that I catch better the reflection from objects suited to the eye at long range than if they were brought too near and the angle of incidence were too acute for proper vision.

In his chapter on The Causal Factors of Amentia, Doctor Tredgold, medical expert to the Royal Commission on the Feebleminded, says: "I believe that ancestral tuberculosis is but rarely the direct and sole cause of amentia; but my observations show that, like alcoholism, it has an important indirect and possibly a contributory influence." He further states: "With regard to persons suffering from amentia, I found a pronounced tendency to tuberculous lesions in the families of thirty-four per cent. of cases investigated." He further states: "There can be no doubt that the death rate from tuberculosis is very much higher (nearly four times as much) in the case of aments than it is in the non-defective population." Now at a first glance these statements would seem to prove beyond dispute that tuberculosis plays a very important contributory if not a directly inciting cause in feeblemindedness. Yet Tredgold states: "It is to be noted, however, that a history of antecedent tuberculosis rarely occurs alone; in four-fifths of my own cases it was accompanied by a definite neuropathic inheritance, while in the remaining fifth, other conditions, usually alcoholism, were also present." It is apparent that statistics on the subject are quite inconclusive, since several possible factors seem to be so commonly present. Recent more exact study inclines to the conclusion that in most Anglo-

* Read at a meeting of the Medical Staff, Otisville Sanatorium.

Saxon communities, whether in Europe or America, the feebleminded of all degrees probably are not less than five per cent in most; yet if the death rate from tuberculosis be put at 0.15 per cent, and the sick from the disease at ten times as many, or 1.5 per cent, in all, we find that there seems statistically no relation between the two. It must have been frequently forced upon the attention of those who have had much to do with the tuberculized, that one of the most obvious conditions present is what for lack of a better term we call a *nerve instability.* I remember that a good many years ago Doctor Mays, of Philadelphia, wrote many articles to prove that tuberculosis was in every sense a disease of the nervous system, and doubtless we have many clinical conditions during the disease in which nervous symptoms play a most important part. Dealing then with the broad aspects of the probable relationship between feeblemindedness and tuberculosis, we have to go back to that subject which has been for years, and is likely to be for years to come, the occasion of much discussion and investigation, viz., the immutability of *germ plasm.* Without entering into the discussion, I wish again to quote what Doctor Tredgold says after a quite full discussion of the subject:

"I hold that primary amentia is a manifestation of a pathological germinal variation which has been produced by the environment, and that the germinal change is of the nature of a vitiation, that is to say, *it consists of an impairment of the intrinsic potentiality for development which may be widespread and affect the germ as a whole or which may be less extensive and confined to the neuronic determinant.* At the beginning in most instances the latter is probably the case and the central change is but slight. It shows itself merely in a diminished function stability and durability of the higher, and therefore an increased excitability of the lower, cerebral neurones and is revealed clinically as neurasthenia, hysteria, migraine, and the milder forms of epilepsy. We may say in fact that these states are the first indications of the presence of the psychopathic diathesis. Should an adverse environment continue, or should a person so affected mate with one similarly tainted, then in the next generation the neuronic durability will be further diminished and the instability accentuated so that insanity, the graver forms of epilepsy, and early dementia make their appearance. If the process is further continued, the third generation will often be characterized by a tendency to defects of anatomical structure, and there will be a strong probability of one or more of the offspring suffering from amentia. Should this germinal impairment be accompanied by any untoward circumstances during the growth of the embryo, this probability will become a tolerable certainty. Degeneracy is here well established and the well-known stigmata indicative of an extensive germinal charge, are usually abundant.

Finally, a condition of gross idiocy appears with complete sterility, and the family becomes extinct."

The breadth of Tredgold's observations and the obviously sane and practical conclusions drawn, make them a convenient basis upon which anything I may say will be based. We all know of mountain valleys in Europe or old-time settlements in America where through intermarriage has been transmitted at times a general cretinism or a general feeblemindedness so marked as to give their people special historic characteristics. The story of the Martin Kallikak family, so well worked out by Goddard, illustrates the fact, and others of us doubtless know family heredity strains quite as marked although not so well worked out statistically. It is *a priori* quite remarkable that in every work dealing with what we may especially term social diseases, as distinct from the acute infectious, viz., tuberculosis, alcoholism, syphilis and feeblemindedness, we find them so often intermingled that it seems quite impossible to determine which disease is the determinant or dominant one. For instance, I recall the history of a family, many of whose members have been known to me, and about whom speaking thirty years ago with my father, we together in a few minutes counted eighty persons who had shown insanity of a catatonic type with mild delusions and periodical acute manifestations. The lists extended back through five generations known either to my father or myself. They were a family many of whom were noted for their beauty, having delicate complexions with golden hair, but in whom the neurotic manifestations were marked especially by mental instability and in a number of cases were associated with consumption. Speaking generally, the mentality of the various branches of the family was more than usually good, and in two distinct branches, descended from brothers intermarried in the second generations with strong stocks of different races, in two instances produced most favorable results in the fourth generation, in the offspring of two second cousins of the fourth generation who intermarried. In all except the last offspring, the fourth generations were country or village bred. We may hence fairly assume that the new blood and good rural surroundings have been building directly toward a neuronic stability, while had the high tension or urban life been allowed to exert its ordinary influence, the departure from the normal would continue. It is interesting to compare this family with the Kallikak family whose history is given with so much accuracy in Goddard's book. In this group the cases starting from a low type under adverse physical environment continue on the same or even a descending plane; but in all cases we revert to the same old question: What is the real underlying cause or causes of the phenomena in any given group of cases? Goddard states that of 1,200 cases of feeblemindedness in the Royal Albert Asylum, phthisis is mentioned in 291 families, or twenty-four per cent of the whole; but no evidence is given that the phthisis present in the children in these families was the cause of feeblemindedness. No class analysis evidently was made through an attempt to go further in these cases. In 327 cases whose family histories have been studied by Goddard, we get a very interesting analysis made:

1. Certain heredity: 164, or 54 per cent—many relatives feebleminded.

2. Probable heredity: 34, or 11.3 per cent—some relatives.

3. Neuropathic ancestry: 37, or 12 per cent—family histories showed various brain affections, from apoplexy to blindness.

4. Accidental cases, 57, or 19 per cent.

5. Unaccounted, 8, or 2.6 per cent.

Speaking of tuberculosis as a causative factor in 324 cases, Goddard points out that cases of tuberculosis are scattered through families in all the four groups and their incidence is such as would be accounted for by contagion. Some of these families show many cases of tuberculosis "due to the low social order of these people," and a recent *Social Survey Report* in Cincinnati says regarding low wages and tenements: "Such a low subsistence level works like black magic in the spread of tuberculosis." After this statement follow notable statistics by Doctor Goddard, which give only 2.8 per cent of all the 324 cases studied as being marked tuberculosis on the chart, while he states the percentage of tuberculized in the general population to be from ten to fifteen per cent. He then draws a somewhat remarkable deduction when he says, "This agrees with the view that feebleminded stock may be primitive and possessed of much animal strength and possibly some immunity from disease." The inference is based upon altogether too limited and imperfect data to be of real value, since we find in actual statistics for over 2,000 school children, that in the children of slum areas, largely British immigrants, the feebleminded are over five per cent of the whole, while the prevalence of tuberculosis has long been known to be directly the measure of bad housing. As I have written elsewhere and as all other sanitary and social works have observed, "tuberculosis is a disease of house life, not the disease of the pioneer shack town; it is the pest of the densely populated city with its slums, overcrowded work rooms and factories." Remembering that the statistics do not note more than "the most clearly defined cases of tuberculosis of the lungs," as Doctor Goddard states, and as we further note that the great proportion of the feebleminded cases examined will have been among children in whom consumption is rare compared with other forms of tuberculosis, I think it may be taken for granted that we can draw but few definite conclusions from these data. The study of Goddard's cases shows much the same with regard to alcohol and leads him to the general conclusion that "everything seems to indicate that alcoholism itself is only a symptom that for the most part occurs in families where there is some form of neurotic taint, especially feeblemindedness." If the result of the careful examination of the antecedents of the feebleminded cannot associate them either with tuberculosis or with alcohol as the exciting cause, and leads us to infer that the feebleminded are for the most part descended from the feebleminded, we seem to be forced back upon the conundrum posed by Doctor Tredgold when, speaking of Weismann's, Davenport's and others' theory of *immutability of germplasm* which must be assumed to belong to members of the simian family, he says "one cannot help wondering how their descendants evolved into human beings at all," and then goes on to say: "I very much doubt whether the phylogeny of civilized man was ever represented by a phase of evolution comparable with that of mental defect. . . . In short, I regard the germinal variation present in these persons as a pathological one; as being of the nature of a vitiation, which instead of being of spontaneous origin is *really due to negation or diminution of spontaneity*. How, then, is this impairment brought about? I consider it primarily due to the action of the environment."

We are thus brought fairly to the crux of our problem. What are we to understand by environment? We have what we call external environment, which is post-natal. The native from the Arctic circle to the equator in every part of the globe is subject to it. The Ojibway Indians of Champlain's time on the shores of Lake Superior are pictured as almost naked in their sun dances and as living on game, fish and herbs; while the Iroquois had their village and cultivated lands and great tribal federations. Similarly the Tasmanian bushmen of the southern hemisphere remained savages, while the Maoris of New Zealand nearby were a proud and intellectual race with federated organization and well developed ideas of land ownership. Evidently there is much in transmitted qualities in spite of mere climatic environment. On the other hand, if we compare Colonel Oglethorpe's settlements in Georgia of the people of the slums of London placed where the environment was negro slavery, with the thousands of the criminal class shipped to Australia, we must confess to the potential influence of environment both physical and human in each case. Indeed it is this latter to which we must lend our attention. Take city life with its persistent high tension, with its constant attacks upon the nervous system, both through business and pleasure, whether in high finance or in the competition of trade, whether in the pursuit of science or medicine, or even in the charities and other social work. It appears to me that we have to widen our outlook in order to observe the broad effects of modern urban life on the one hand, and on the other to endeavor to realize what internal environment means. Similarly there is *prenatal* environment. We understand the rapidity of cell multiplication and know that there is cell differentiation in the ovum. We further know that from the simplest particle of vital protoplasm through all the stages of cell evolution up to pyramidal brain cells and those of the ductless glands, such depend upon normal nutrition for their growth; while we learn from feeding experiments, as well as investigations into the antecedents of monsters, in animals at birth, of the distinctly injurious effects upon young chicks during incubation of irregular heating, deficient moisture and impure air, as well as of the destructive effects upon the fetus of systematic poisons, whether mineral, as in lead poisoning, or of infectious diseases as in smallpox, which often result in its death. But much more serious because more general are the hammering effects, to use a mechanical term, of urban life upon the nervous system. Every observant physician, taking stock of his female patients, endeavors to remove the prospective mother from an untoward environment when he notices the undue strain upon her nervous system. For multitudes of the poorer class, rest is impossible; but Nature with her resources has often, through habits of labor, supplied the defence of an originally less impressible nervous system with a rugged nutrition, the outcome of physical labor. But to many women the noise, the rush, the excitement in their daily lives results either in a complete nerve exhaustion or in a neurasthenia, though occasionally, in a response of Nature to the demand for an extra output of energy when under physical pain or some great emotion, such as war, an abnormal resistance is developed through the sympathetic nervous system. But it is most true, as expressed by John Martin, that "appealingly common are the cases of girls with these nervous organizations and delicate brains, whose latent maturity has been rendered a torture by the exhaustion following on their conscientious obedience to the demands of school and college, of social work, or society life." The most noticeable gross effects are seen in the general reduction in the birth rate in all progressive countries where urbanization is going on rapidly. Thus Doctor Newsholme, chief medical officer, has estimated that had the birth rate of England and Wales been the same in 1914 as in 1876 there would have been 467,837 more infants born there in 1914 than actually saw the light. In a recent report to the Prussian Diet it was stated that there were 560,000 fewer births in Germany than would have occurred if the birth rate of 1900 had been maintained. It was further declared that the decline in birth rate in Germany in twelve years had been as rapid as that in France in seventy, and that births had dropped seventy-five per cent more than deaths. The most important speakers at the society dealing with the problem pointed out that the cause is essentially economic, the average marriage age for men being now twenty-nine and for women twenty-six years. Earlier marriage was urged as tending to lessen syphilis and illegitimacy. There are 180,000 illegitimate children born every year in Germany. The recognition of the serious effects upon the child, in the prenatal stage, as well as upon the mother, of disease and disturbed mental conditions, is illustrated in the very successful work being done in maternity hospitals through the care of the mother during this period. Thus in thirty-four mothers treated in Edinburgh during three months, seventeen had albuminuria, yet thirty-three were safely delivered; but there were forty-six per cent. of still-births, although eighty per cent. of the mothers were married. The need for antenatal clinics is thus made obvious.

We have thus illustrated the general effects of environment on prenatal health and may now revert to the direct influence of tuberculosis during this period. All will have noted how the progress of tuberculosis often for the time is stayed during pregnancy. Fetal life often greatly stimulates appetite and nutrition in the mother, only to be followed by a complete breakdown during lactation. During gestation, therefore, it may be that the toxic effects of the tuberculous process are lessened or that they may act as an immunizing factor in the child; but the large number of tuberculous cases, where the child apparently becomes inoculated directly from the mother after birth suggests that the amount of antecedent immunization must have been too small. Regarding its direct effects in promoting feeblemindedness, Tredgold, like Goddard, says: "I believe that ancestral tuberculosis is but rarely the direct sole cause of amentia; but my observations show that, like alcoholism, it has an important indirect and possibly a contributory influence. This indirect effect is seen in its potency to produce the milder and initial forms of nervous instability in the offspring such as migraine, hysteria and neurasthenia, a clinical fact which has been frequently noticed." It is very remarkable how in the works of the two great authorities on amentia cited, each constantly turns to the condition of neuronic instability which finds its daily illustration and expression in the effects of modern urbanization. Let any family physician declare his experience, and he will tell that his chief energies are spent upon patching up systems where there is anemia, malnutrition, functional disturbance of organs, inability to perform normal duties, and where some nerve whip or tonic is frequently required, much of this condition soon disappearing with rest under changed environment as at some rest cure. In many of this class certain common symptoms are observable, such as an actual dislike or even physical distress at the appearance of the older coarse forms of food such as fats, oatmeal and so on, and a longing for sweet or spiced foods which excite appetite or stimulate the gustatory nerves. Indeed it is abundantly plain that the food of the well-to-do in America is very different from that of the sturdy immigrant peasant, whether Russian, Austrian or Italian, while it is very probable that among the other vices of our civilization, that of an irrational dietary and of foods of imperfect nutritive elements due to the robbing our common foods, as the grains, of their salts and vitamines is not the least important. What we are assured of is that though the protective measures against the direct attacks of tuberculosis and other infectious diseases are being constantly multiplied by science and official supervision, yet the breaking down of the *nerve* defences proceeds constantly through the thousand and one modern influences hammering at our brain through the special senses, such as noises, "movies," and the dissipating effects of abnormal occupations and of irregular hours, which exhaust the physical powers and the ability to resist degenerative or malign causes operating against the normal physical and mental processes. We have observed the phenomenon of how in almost every country, certainly in North America, the urban population of fifty years ago was but twenty-five per cent. of the total, while in the United States and Canada at least fifty per cent. of the total population is to-day urbanized in cities of 5,000 or over, while probably twenty-five per cent. more are suburbanites and in small villages and towns, leaving but twenty-five per cent. actually engaged in agriculture. The effects of the change upon two succeeding generations are now becoming apparent, and we are seriously asking ourselves whether phylogeny will disappear in its old normal developmental influences, to be replaced by some modern man-created eugenics, adequate to cope with the changed environment, including habits of life, housing, occupation and education. We know that our total death rate, as in New York, has been cut in two in fifty years; but we likewise know that the saving is due almost solely to the application of what we may term artificial methods. To give some instances:

1. We have enormously limited the birth rate, leaving, we are told, just so much more time to care for the newborn.

2. The nursing mother has, however, almost disappeared, while much more time is occupied in the attempts to make the child of the neurotic mother, with its hypersensitive nerve reflexes of the digestive organs, digest artificially prepared foods.

3. The child with no green pastures to run in beside the still waters, is at best conveyed from the flat to the nearest park by the typical nurse

girl, although, indeed, most urban children are born and bred in the tenement and suffer from all its limitations.

4. The mental environment is artificial under all these conditions, and in northern climates the limitations caused by six months or more of our modern housing have produced and will produce a type which as Dr. Creighton Browne says, "is distinctly more jumpy than we used to be."

5. My observations and the teachings of psychology based on physiology make it apparent that with the absence of a Nature environment at a time when the special senses are absolutely normal in their ability to receive impressions, the growth of mind, based upon artificial environment, will make it more difficult for each succeeding urban generation to wish to get back or to absorb normally, even were the wish present, those elementary Nature impressions which are still the underlying basis of the thoughts of the modern generation. Whether or not modern social processes will develop their physiological or patholgical immunizing changes needed to meet the new life conditions being so rapidly developed under modern peace and war times, as regards urbanization, inventions and artificial products of every sort, must remain to the future for proof. Meantime the degeneration of tissue or the wearing out process has become statistically recognized even in slow-going England, while every hospital, sanatorium, asylum, refuge and "home"—and their class is ever increasing—is filled with the casualties due to this modern war against normal natural processes.

The following table showing the growth of hospitals and patients in the Province of Ontario is both instructive and hortatory:

	Total Hospitals in Ontario	Total Patients	Total Population of Province	Ratio of Patients in Population
1880	12	5,237	1,926,922	1 in 369
1890	24	10,523	2,114,321	1 " 200
1900	52	29,761	2,189,947	1 " 72
1908	60	46,971	2,280,359	1 " 48
1910	78	53,692	2,523,274	1 " 47
1915	91	85,759	2,598,320	1 " 30

If by any artificial methods we may greatly limit tuberculosis, we still have a problem of feeblemindedness to attack, which will, for an unknown period under modern life conditions, give our legislators, educationists, clerics and physicians ample occupation if they are to solve the problem satisfactorily.

Date Due

MEDICAL

616.9955
N533t

New York. Dept. Health
Bryce
Tuberculosis in relation to feeblemindedness

Betty Moledy
353 Best

3/24 MAR

UNIVERSITY OF MICHIGAN

3 9015 04553 4933

PUBLICATIONS

OF THE

DEPARTMENT OF HEALTH OF THE CITY OF NEW YORK

Monthly Bulletin. Established in January, 1911. The Bulletin contains summary tables of vital statistics for the preceding month, together with descriptive articles and notes intended for the instruction of the public and for the information of physicians and others concerned in public health work.

Weekly Bulletin. This contains a weekly summary of vital statistics and brief public health news of current interest. At the present time, only a small edition of reprints is available for mailing to public health officials and others particularly interested.

Monthly Drug Bulletin. A monthly publication which aims to enlist the co-operation of druggists in public health work by presenting to them an account of those activities of the Department of Health which pertain largely to their own work. This bulletin is mailed, without charge, to all drug stores in the city.

School Health News. A monthly publication designed to secure the co-operation of school teachers in the work of the Department of Health. This publication is sent to each school, in quantity sufficient to supply each teacher with one copy. There is no mailing list for individual teachers.

Neighborhood Health Chronicles. These are simply written, popular leaflets, published monthly for the purpose of instructing the masses in health matters. They are prepared in co-operation with local health agencies, and are distributed directly into the homes. There is no mailing list.

Staff News. A monthly publication for the instruction of employes of the Department of Health. It contains both news items and official notices and orders. This publication is distributed only to those connected with the Department of Health.

Collected Studies from the Research Laboratory. An annual collection of scientific papers presenting the work done at the bacteriological laboratories for the year.

Monograph Series. A series of special papers by officials or employes of the Department, each dealing with some particular problem or phase of the Department's work. These papers appear from time to time, ' no specified interval.

Reprint Series. The Department occasionally reprints at i' expense and distributes shorter papers published by its o' employes in medical and other scientific journals. Such published in a standard serial form, with a list of thos' distribution.

Tuberculosis Monographs. This consists of scien' with various phases of tuberculosis. There is r but the publication will be sent on request to t'

Other Publications. The Department of H ous pamphlets of rules and regulations, r tions and advice to public on particul' classified or listed.

TUBERCULOSIS MONOGRAPHS

No. 1. A Study on Food and the Food Value of the Dietary at the New York City Municipal Sanatorium. By Robert J. Wilson, M.D., Director of the Bureau of Hospitals, Department of Health, and Walter L. Rathbun, M.D., Physician-in-Charge, New York City Municipal Sanatorium.

No. 2. Laryngeal Tuberculosis: A Three Years' Study. By Julius Dworetzky, M.D., New York City Municipal Sanatorium.

No. 3. Tuberculosis in Relation to Feeblemindedness. By Peter Bryce, M.A., M.D., Chief Medical Officer of the Interior, and Chief Medical Inspector of Immigration for Canada.

The Department will enter into exchange of publications with public health, medical and scientific organizations, societies, laboratories, journals and authors. Applications for publications should be addressed to the Bureau of Public Health Education, Department of Health, 139 Centre Street, New York City.

www.ingramcontent.com/pod-product-compliance
Lightning Source LLC
LaVergne TN
LVHW010834120826
845149LV00016B/1377